DIAGNOSTIC PIC

D1644587

Sexually Transmitted Diseases

Patrick K Taylor FRCOG
Consultant in Genito-Urinary Medicine
Bristol Royal Infirmary
Bristol BS2 8HW, England

M Mosby-Wolfe

London Baltimore Bogotá Boston Buenos Aires Caracas Carlsbad, CA Chicago Madrid Mexico City Milan Naples, FL
New York Philadelphia St. Louis Sydney Tokyo Toronto Wiesbaden

Titles published in the Diagnostic Picture Tests series include:

Picture Tests in Human Anatomy	DPT in Cardiology
DPT in Clinical Medicine, Vol 1–4	DPT in Clinical Neurology
DPT in Dermatology	DPT in Ear, Nose and Throat
DPT in Embryology	DPT in Endocrinology
DPT in Gastroenterology	DPT in General Dentistry
DPT in General Medicine	DPT in General Surgery
DPT in Geriatric Medicine	DPT in Infectious Diseases
DPT in Differential Diagnosis in AIDS	DPT in Injury in Sport
DPT in Obstetrics and Gynaecology	DPT in Ophthalmology
DPT in Oral Medicine Orthopaedics	DPT in Paediatrics, 2nd edition
DPT in Paediatric Dentistry	DPT in Respiratory Disease
DPT in Rheumatology	DPT in Urology

400 Self-Assesment Picture Tests in Clinical Medicine
400 More Self-Assesment Picture Tests in Clinical Medicine

Copyright © 1995 Times Mirror International Publishers Limited

Published in 1995 by Mosby-Wolfe, an imprint of Times Mirror International Publishers Limited

Project Manager Roderick Craig

Publisher Richard Furn

Production Mike Heath

Printed in Spain by Grafos, S.A. ARTE SOBRE PAPEL

ISBN 0 7234 1965 5

All rights reserved. No part of this publication may be reproduced, stored in a retrieval system, copied or transmitted, in any form or by any means, electronic, mechanical, photocopying, recording or otherwise without written permission from the Publisher or in accordance with the provisions of the Copyright Act 1956 (as amended), or under the terms of any licence permitting limited copying issued by the Copyright Licensing Agency, 33–34 Alfred Place, London, WC1E 7DP.

Any person who does any unauthorised act in relation to this publication may be liable to criminal prosecution and civil claims for damages.

Permission to photocopy or reproduce solely for internal or personal use is permitted for libraries or other users registered with the Copyright Clearance Center, provided that the base fee of $4.00 per chapter plus $.10 per page is paid directly to the Copyright Clearance Center, 21 Congress Street, Salem, MA 01970. This consent does not extend to other kinds of copying, such as copying for general distribution, for advertising or promotional purposes, for creating new collected works, or for resale.

For full details of all Times Mirror International Publishers Limited titles, please write to Times Mirror International Publishers Limited, Lynton House, 7–12 Tavistock Square, London WC1H 9LB, England.

A CIP catalogue record for this book is available from the British Library.

Library of Congress Cataloging-in-Publication Data applied for.

Acknowledgements

Production of this book would not have been possible without the generous help of the many friends and colleagues who have allowed me to use their slides. I would like to thank the following for their permission to reproduce photographs:
Dr A N McClean (figures 20, 89, 134, 144, 145, 148, 149, 162 & 163); Dr J Arumainayagam (figures 27, 39, 40, 135, 136, 186, 197, 198 & 199); Dr S Norman (figures 17, 18, 23, 41, 64–6, 75–6, 88, 91–3, 113–14, 116, 124, 137, 164–5, 171, 190–91 & 193); the late Dr A E Tinkler (figures 69 & 138). I am also grateful to Mosby-Wolfe for the use of figures 10, 19, 34, 48, 58, 79, 83, 87, 104, 118–19, 139 & 168–9 from *A Colour Atlas of Sexually Transmitted Diseases* by Dr Anthony Wisdom, and figures 57, 100, 128, 147, 177 & 188–9 from *A Colour Atlas of AIDS* by Dr Charles Farthing et al.
Finally I should like to thank Miss E Hurst and her colleagues in the Department of Medical Illustration at the Bristol Royal Infirmary for their invaluable help in producing the slides.

Preface

Although this book is not a textbook, I have attempted to include in it a wide variety of patients who have attended Genito-Urinary Medicine departments over the past few years. Many of the cases are common, everyday examples but I have also included some rare presentations. The work of GU Medicine encompasses a wide sphere of activity and I hope that perhaps by reading this book and attempting to answer the questions, someone may be tempted to enter the speciality. Senior students and those studying for higher examinations should find the book helpful.

Patrick Taylor

1 What is this condition of the scrotum?

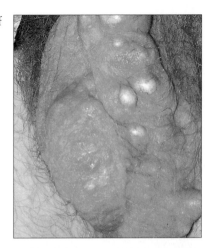

2 (a) Which disease causes this typical painless lesion?
(b) What is its correct name?
(c) What other helpful clinical sign is invariably present?

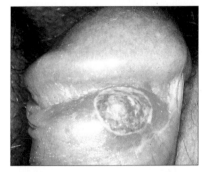

3 This 19-year-old youth developed a urethral discharge and mild dysuria two days after a casual sexual encounter.
(a) What is the most likely diagnosis?
(b) List the other pathological causes of urethral discharge.

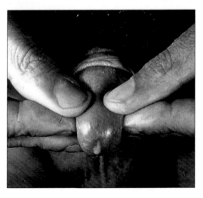

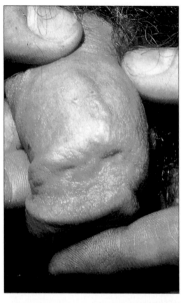

4 A patient attends with this firm, worm-like lesion of his penis.
(a) What is the lesion?
(b) How is it caused?
(c) What is the treatment?

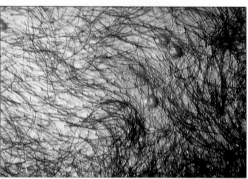

5 (a) What are these lesions?
(b) In what condition are they commonly found on the face?

6 (a) What does this radio-graph show in a young man?
(b) What is its common name?
(c) In what conditions is it found?

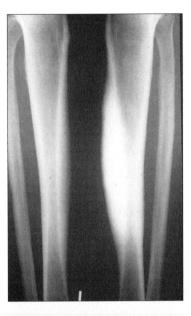

7 A young man was seen after several weeks' treatment with podophyllin to these 'coronal warts' proved ineffective. What are they?

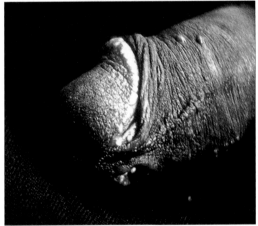

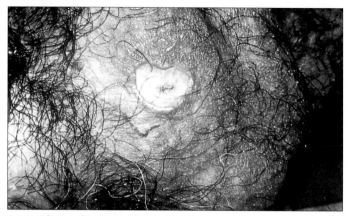

8 (a) What is the cause of this painful scrotal sore associated with aphthous ulceration?
(b) In which regions of the world is it most common?
(c) What other conditions must be excluded?

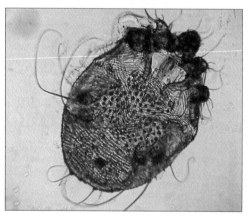

9 (a) What is this ectoparasite?
(b) In which layer of the skin is it found?

10 This asymptomatic lesion of the tongue was found in a 32-year-old homosexual man with AIDS-related-complex.
(a) What is the lesion?
(b) Which virus, apart from HIV, is thought to be implicated in its causation?

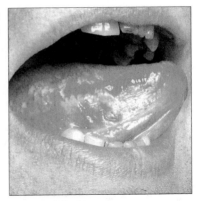

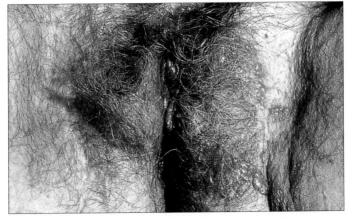

11 A 40-year-old woman developed this condition, which was preceded by localised pain.
(a) What is the diagnosis?
(b) How does its distribution distinguish it from a common related condition?

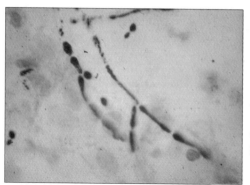

12 (a) What does this Gram-stained slide show?
(b) At what pH and on what culture medium is it most commonly grown?

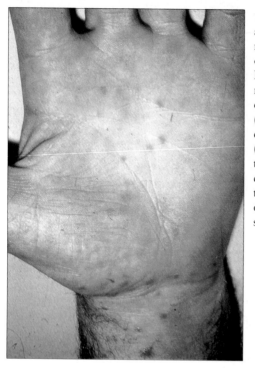

13 A patient attended with a non-pruritic rash on her trunk. Examination also revealed this rash on her palms.
(a) What is the diagnosis?
(b) Which other two sites in the distribution of the rash are often of help in diagnosis?

14, 15 A 35-year-old man presented with painful swelling of his left knee and ankle together with this painless penile rash.
(a) What is wrong with him?
(b) What is the rash known as?

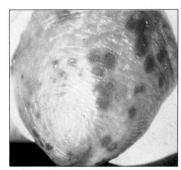

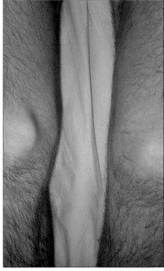

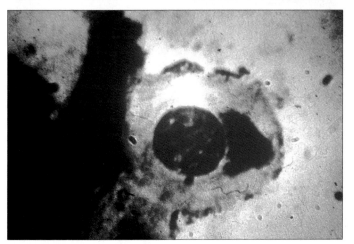

16 (a) What does this picture show?
(b) What conditions are caused by this organism in the neonate?

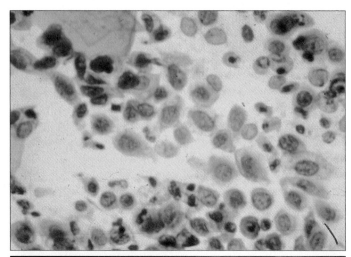

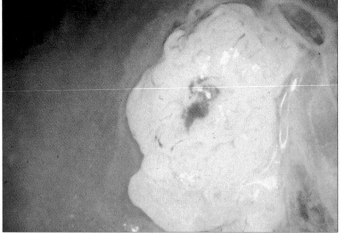

17, 18 A woman had a cervical cytology and was advised to return for colposcopy. She said she would have one in Australia as she was leaving the following day. When she returned a year later, having failed to arrange this examination, she had developed a lesion on her cervix.

(a) What did the cytology show?

(b) What is the lesion?

19 What does this smear show?

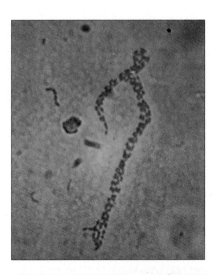

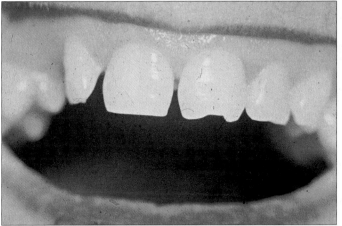

20 (a) What is this condition of the incisor teeth and its cause?
(b) In which disease does it occur?
(c) What other dental abnormality is sometimes found in this condition?

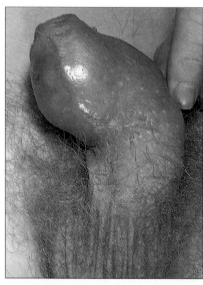

21 This man's penis assumed the characteristic shape of a musical instrument.
(a) What is the instrument giving the lesion its eponym?
(b) What is the cause of the condition?

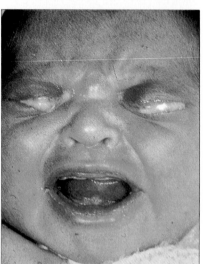

22 (a) What is this condition contracted during birth?
(b) What organisms might be responsible?
(c) How would you manage the problem?

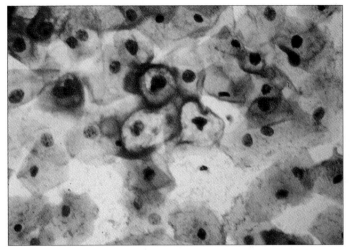

23 (a) What are the predominant cells in this cervical cytology smear?
(b) What is their significance?

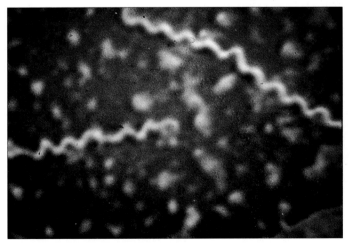

24 (a) What is this organism?
(b) By what method is it demonstrated in this picture?

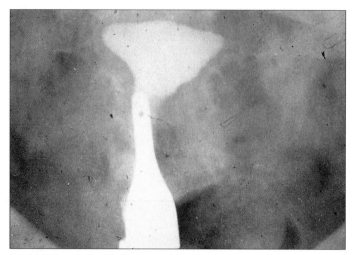

25 (a) What does this hysterosalpingogram show on a young woman being investigated for infertility?
(b) What is the likely predisposing cause?
(c) What technique is now more usually employed to demonstrate this condition?

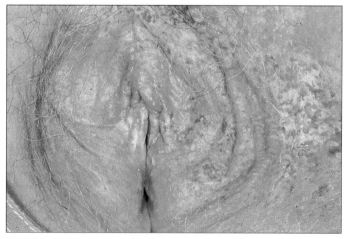

26 What is the cause of this irritant, scaly, erythematous plaque found in a 44-year-old lady?

27 This chest radiograph in a patient with AIDS shows early lung involvement with Kaposi's sarcoma. What other non-infectious cause of lung disease is often seen in patients with AIDS?

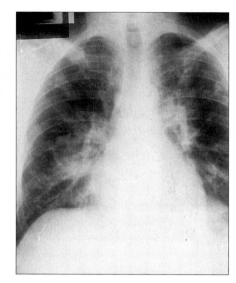

28 This woman suffered from a greyish, muco-purulent vaginal discharge. No infective cause was found and the condition improved after she stopped taking her oral contraceptive. Why?

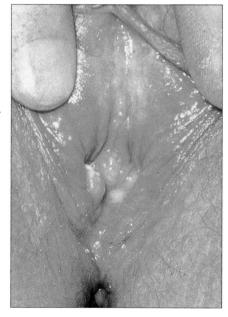

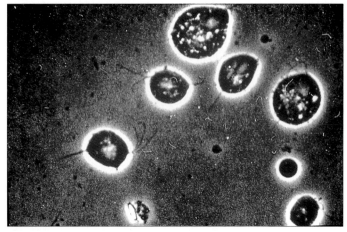

29 (a) These motile organisms are a common source of vaginal infection. What are they?
(b) What is the drug of choice in their treatment?

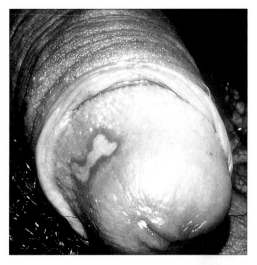

30 (a) What are these ulcers associated with painful inguinal lymphadeno-pathy?
(b) How would you confirm the diagnosis?

31 A 25-year-old woman presented with these vulval lesions.
(a) What are they?
(b) With what systemic disease are they associated?
(c) In which other areas of the body may they occur?
(d) How are they treated?

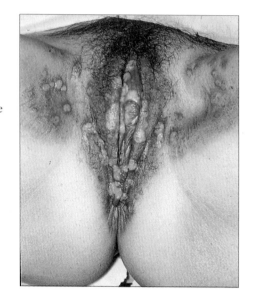

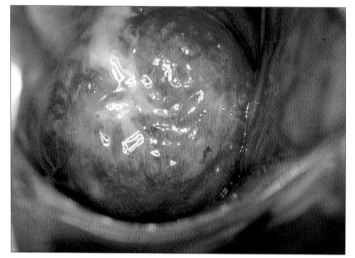

32 (a) What does this picture show?
(b) List some common causes.

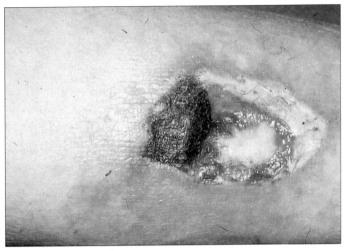

33 (a) What is this ulcer?
(b) What is its base often described as looking like?
(c) How does its distribution on the leg differ from a varicose ulcer?

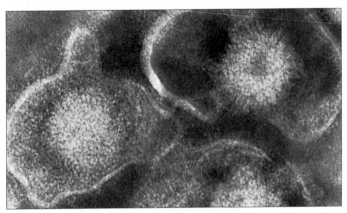

34 (a) Which common virus does this electron photomicrograph show ?
(b) The phenomenon of latency occurs with this virus. Where is the virus found at this time?

35 (a) What classic triad of symptoms of Reiter's disease includes this condition?
(b) In what percentage of patients with non-gonococcal urethritis does Reiter's disease occur?
(c) What other cause acts as a trigger for reactive arthritis?

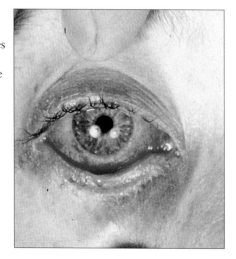

36 This patient stole the medication being used to treat his warts twice weekly in the clinic and proceded to apply it himself twice daily. This resulted in the blistering and burns shown.
(a) What is the likely agent involved?
(b) What other common methods are used to treat genital warts?

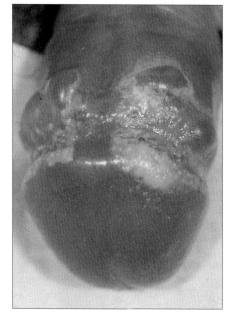

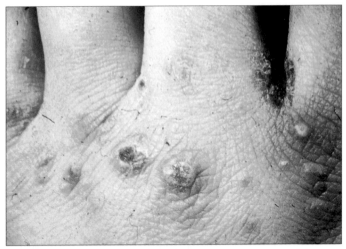

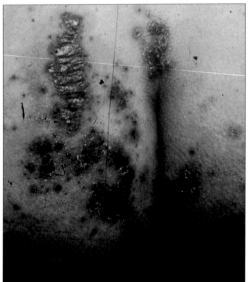

37, 38 What are these lesions on the fingers and buttocks of a young man who also had an intensely irritant rash on his abdomen, which became worse at night?

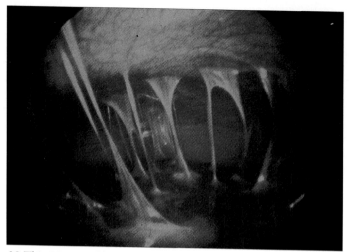

39 This 23-year-old woman presented with severe upper right quadrant abdominal pain, which followed a mild lower abdominal aching one week previously. Laparoscopy was performed.
(a) What did laparoscopy reveal?
(b) What is the diagnosis?
(c) What organisms may be responsible?
(d) What is the differential diagnosis?

40 A 29-year-old woman with HIV infection presented with symptoms of dysphagia and pain on swallowing.
(a) What did endoscopy show?
(b) What is the treatment of choice?
(c) What side effects can occur as a result of this treatment?
(d) What other conditions can cause dysphagia in HIV infection?

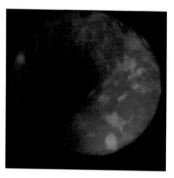

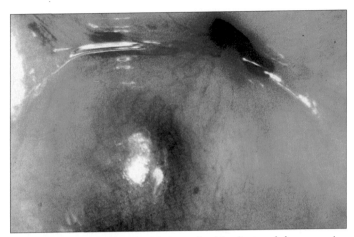

41 This patient presented with irregular bleeding and dyspareunia. What does colposcopy show?

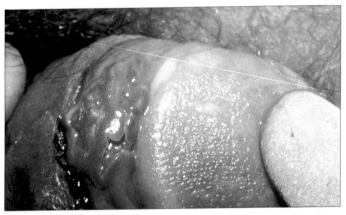

42 This 28-year-old man has just returned from Africa, where he had visited a prostitute. This painful sore occurred one week after exposure.

(a) What is the diagnosis?

(b) What are the causative organisms?

(c) How are these demonstrated?

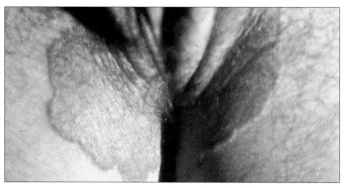

43 (a) What is this irritant rash found on a 26-year-old lorry driver?
(b) Which organisms are commonly involved and at which other sites are they commonly found?
(c) What is the differential diagnosis?

44 (a) What is this typical appearance of the vagina due to?
(b) What symptoms would the patient be likely to experience?

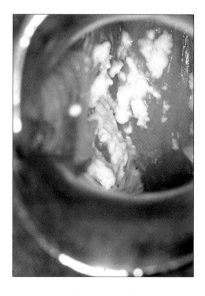

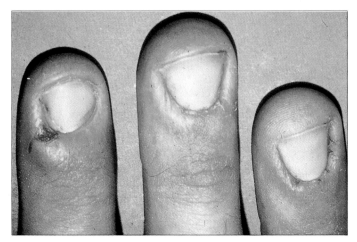

45 (a) How was this herpetic paronychia probably contracted?
(b) Which other extra-genital sites may be infected in the same way?

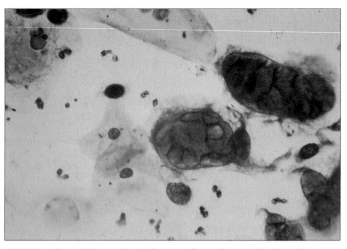

46 What does this cytological smear from the cervix show?

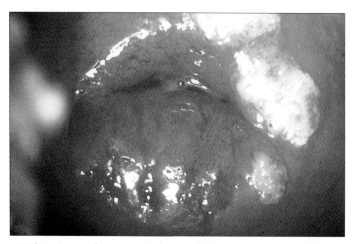

47 This picture shows cervical warts following treatment with trichloracetic acid. What common subtypes of human papilloma virus are found in genital lesions?

48 A Gram-stained smear was taken from a woman with a yellow, odorous, frothy vaginal discharge.
(a) What does it show?
(b) By what name is the condition now generally known?
(c) How is it treated?

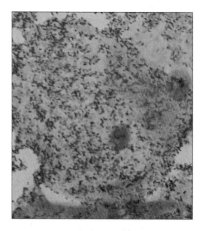

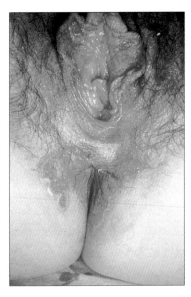

49 A young woman attended the clinic complaining of loss of scalp hair after suffering a mild throat infection. Examination revealed these vulval lesions.
(a) What is the diagnosis?
(b) What will happen to her hair?

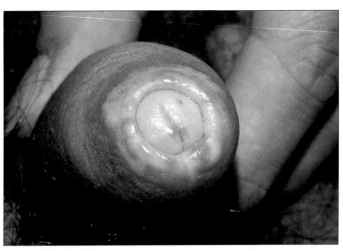

50 (a) What is this progressive condition?
(b) What complication is developing here?
(c) How is it treated?
(d) In women it manifests itself as what condition?

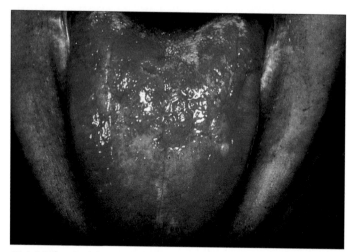

51 (a) What is this tongue lesion in a man with late syphilis who complained of discomfort on eating hot or spicy foods?
(b) What may happen in this condition?

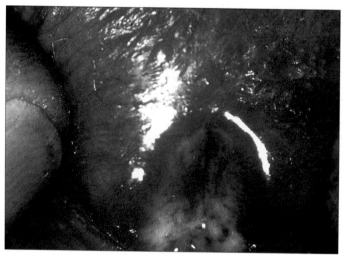

52 This man complained of recurrent attacks of severe dysuria and mucoid urethral discharge every three months. Investigation of his urine was always negative.
What is the cause if his symptoms?

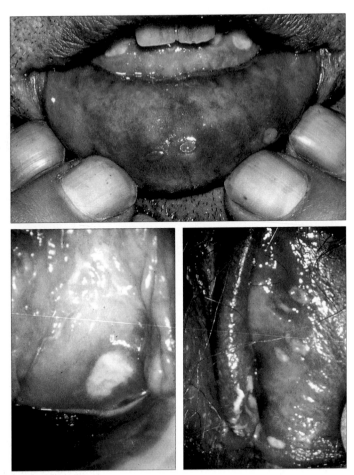

53, 54, 55 These recurrent lesions of the mouth, vaginal vault and labia have been present in the patient for several years. She has now presented with uveitis. There is no sexually transmitted infection.

(a) What is the diagnosis?

(b) What other systemic symptoms might be found?

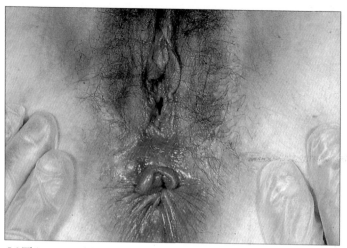

56 This perianal lesion was found in a female patient.
(a) What is the probable diagnosis?
(b) Where else would one look for evidence of infection?
(c) What is this lesion often mistaken for?

57 A man with AIDS presented with severe, watery, painless diarrhoea.
(a) What does this Ziehl-Nielsen staining of a stool specimen show?
(b) What other causes of diarrhoea are definitive of AIDS infection?

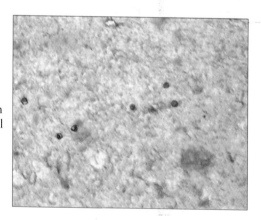

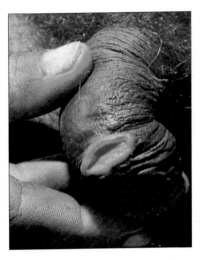

58 (a) What is this, now rare, penile lesion with a typical rolled edge presenting in a 60-year-old West Indian man?

(b) Similar scrotal lesions used to be an occupational hazard in which jobs?

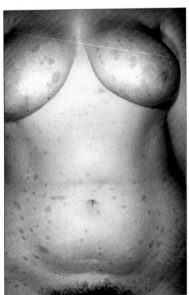

59 This patient was referred with a diagnosis of secondary syphilis. However, she gave a history of a larger, irritant solitary red lesion that had appeared ten days previously, and her present rash was also mildly itchy.

(a) What is the diagnosis?

(b) What was the initial lesion?

(c) What is the treatment?

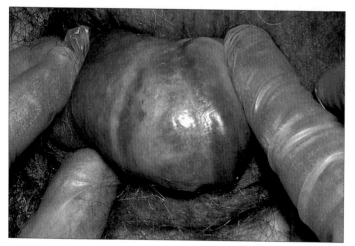

60 This patient purchased some cream in a sex shop that would allegedly increase his pleasure when lovemaking. It caused quite the opposite. What has happened?

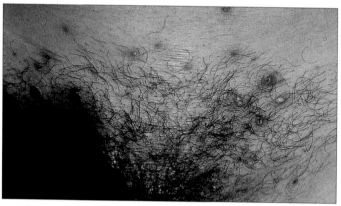

61 This patient with scabies scratched his lesions and caused another problem.
(a) What is it?
(b) What is the cause of the rash in scabies?

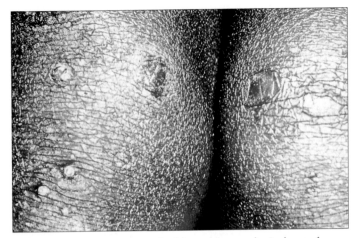

62 This young man presented with positive serological tests for syphilis. These scars were noted on his knees. When questioned, it was discovered that he had been treated for a non-venereal treponematosis in the West Indies.

(a) What did he have?

(b) What other non-venereal treponematoses are found in tropical areas?

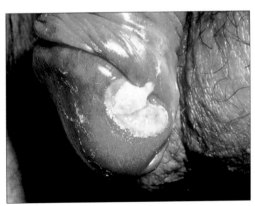

63 What are these irregular crusted penile lesions?

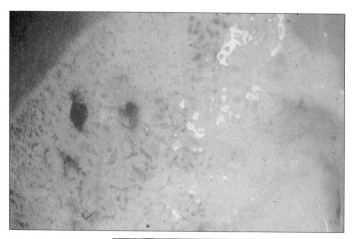

64, 65, 66 These three pictures show the colposcopic, cytological and histological appearance of the same condition.
(a) What is the diagnosis?
(b) Describe the cytological appearance.
(c) Who created the stain commonly used for cervical cytology?

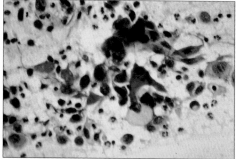

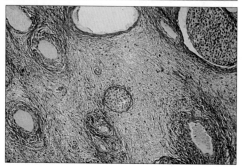

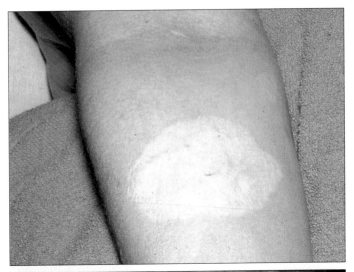

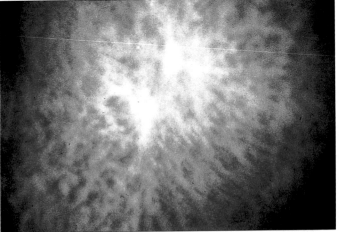

67, 68 The scarring shown is typical of the healing process in two different conditions. Name the condition and type of scarring in each case.

69 (a) What does this urethrogram show?
(b) What infection is likely to have caused the problem?

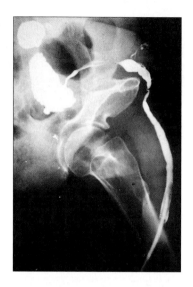

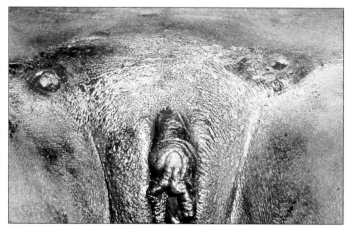

70 This woman, recently arrived from the Caribbean, presented with discharging bilateral inguinal lymph nodes associated with malaise and mild pyrexia.
(a) What is the likely diagnosis?
(b) What is the differential diagnosis?

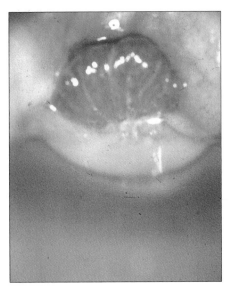

71 What is this cervical lesion in a woman with post-coital and inter-menstrual bleeding?

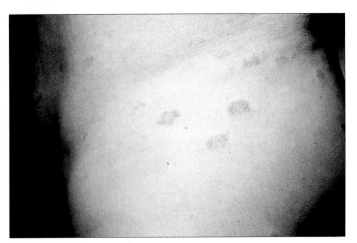

72 What are these itchy areas on this patient's trunk?

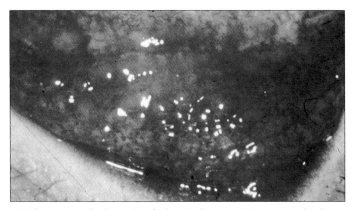

73 This patient had a gritty feeling in her eye. Her partner had a urethral discharge.
(a) What is the eye infection?
(b) Different serotypes of the same organisms cause one of the world's most common forms of blindness. What is the disease?

74 This 17-year-old prostitute was contacted following a client's visit to the clinic. She was unaware that there was anything wrong with her.
(a) What is the diagnosis?
(b) What is the normal incubation period?
(c) What should the patient be warned about that might occur a few hours after commencing treatment?
(d) What is the name for this?

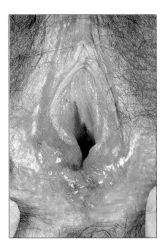

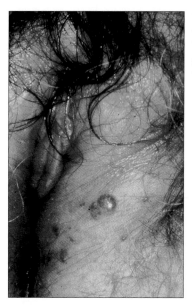

75 This small vulval lump was thought by the patient to be malignant. She was reassured that it was benign. What is it?

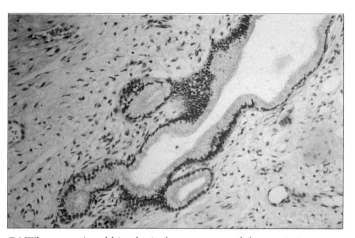

76 What occasional histological appearance of the cervix is shown?

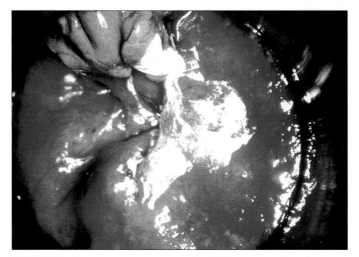

77 (a) What is seen on proctoscopy in this homosexual patient presenting with anal dampness and discomfort?
(b) List the causes of this condition in this group of patients.

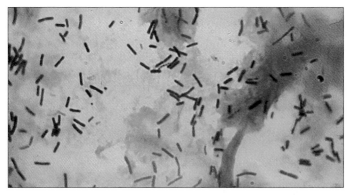

78 These Gram-positive organisms are part of the normal flora of the vagina.
(a) What are they?
(b) What is their function?
(c) How do they achieve this?

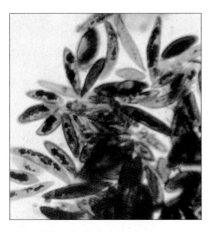

79 (a) Which opportunistic infection by trophozoites is shown?
(b) What is the commonest presentation of trophozoite infection in patients with AIDS?

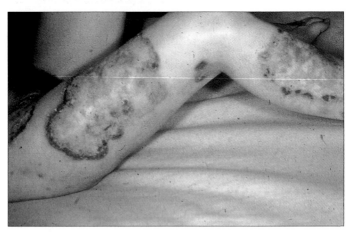

80 This patient has an extensive progressive lesion showing darkly pigmented areas of activity and hypopigmented healed areas.
(a) Of what is this a typical appearance?
(b) What is the treatment?

81, 82 These itchy, violaceous papules on the penis of a 35-year-old man were associated with a white latticework inside his cheek.
(a) What is the diagnosis?
(b) What is the network of fine white lines over the surface of the penile lesions called?

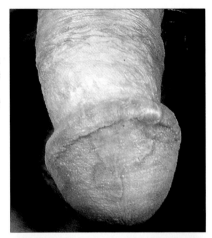

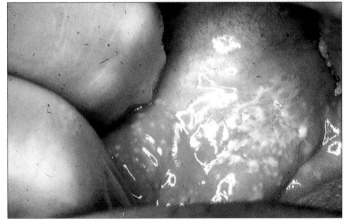

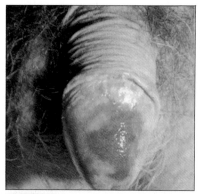

83 (a) What is this sharply demarcated, velvety-red, glistening lesion found in a 55-year-old man?
(b) What would you expect on biopsy?

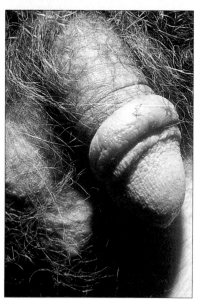

84 (a) What is this local complication of herpes simplex infection?
(b) List the other complications of herpes.

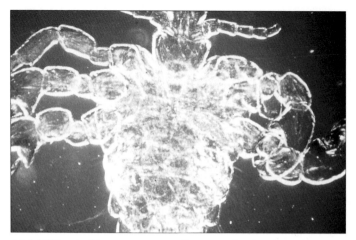

85 (a) What is this common sexually-transmitted arthropod?
(b) What other similar species are seen in humans?
(c) What infections may they transmit?

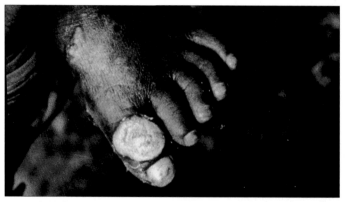

86 A child from Trinidad had this lesion on his foot due to a non-venereal treponematosis.
(a) What is the lesion?
(b) What is the causative organism?
(c) How is it transmitted?

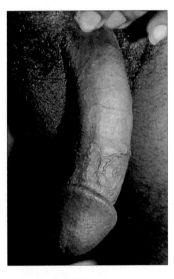

87 A 42-year-old man complains of pain and deviation of his penis to one side on erection.
(a) What is this condition?
(b) What other sign is shown in this picture?
(c) With what other connective tissue disorder is it sometimes associated?

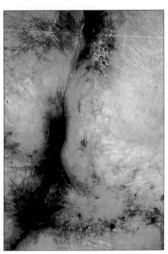

88 This woman with a persistently sore vulva eventually had a colposcopic examination. Biopsy showed vulval intra-epithelial neoplasia. With what dystrophic disorder is this associated?

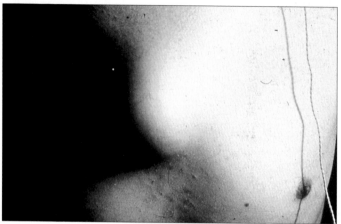

89, 90 This mass on the anterior chest wall of one patient and a chest radiograph of another patient with a similar condition illustrate a complication found in a small percentage of patients with syphilis.

(a) What is the condition?

(b) What characteristic would you expect the mass to have?

(c) What other manifestations can syphilis produce when this body system is affected?

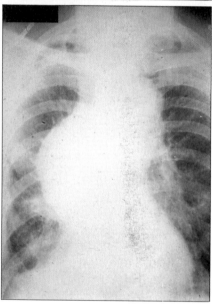

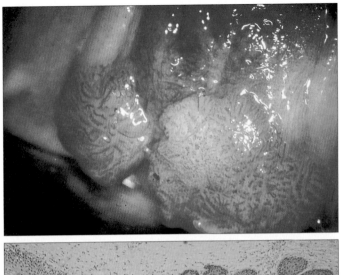

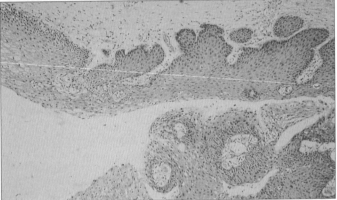

91, 92 A patient attended with post-coital bleeding. What is the cause of her symptoms, confirmed by biopsy?

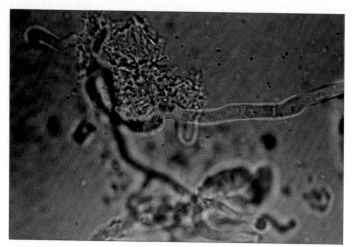

93 What is this method of demonstrating fungal skin infections?

94 This 10-year-old girl presented with soreness of her vulva and a slight discharge that her mother noticed on her daughter's underclothes.
(a) What is the differential diagnosis?
(b) How was the condition acquired?

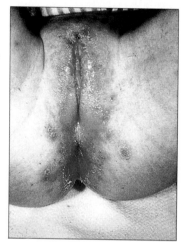

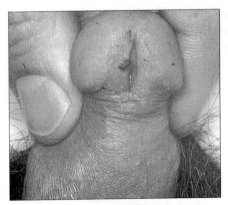

95 (a) What is this congenital abnormality of the penis?
(b) What is the pigmented lesion shown?

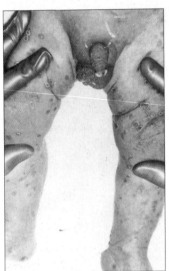

96 A baby with congenital syphilis developed this rash four weeks after birth.
(a) How would you confirm the diagnosis?
(b) Does a bullous rash ever occur in syphilis?
(c) Describe the primary chancre in congenital syphilis.

97 What is this, now rare, painful swelling of the penis associated with urethritis?

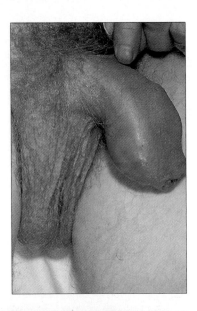

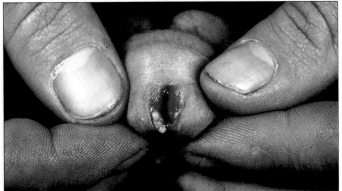

98 This patient complained of bleeding from his urethra. Examination revealed the cause of his symptoms.
(a) What was the cause?
(b) What other conditions might have been responsible?

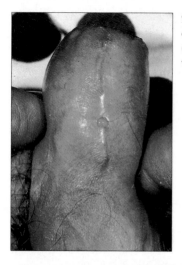

99 (a) What is this lesion found on the ventral penile surface? (b) Is infection ever associated with it?

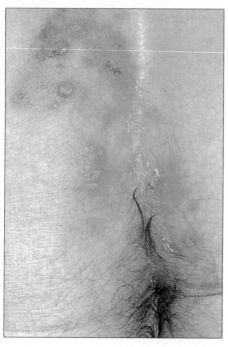

100 (a) Severe peri-anal manifestations of this infection are commonly seen in which condition? (b) What is the infection?

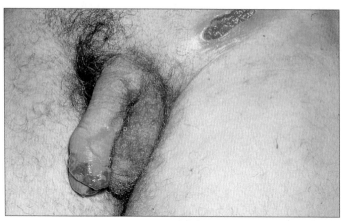

101, 102 (a) What is this condition seen in an immigrant from Africa?
(b) What is the cause of the condition?
(c) The diagnosis is often helped by which feature illustrated?

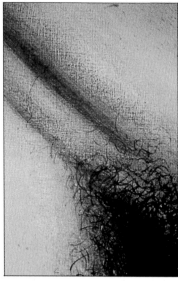

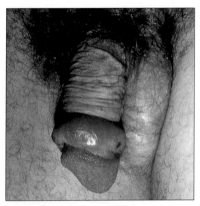

103 (a) What is this condition?
(b) How is it caused?
(c) What is the treatment?

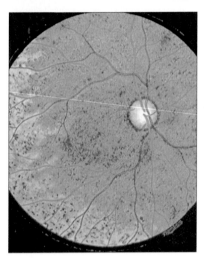

104 This condition is often found as a result of early damage in congenital syphilis.
(a) What is it?
(b) How is it often described?

105 This colpo-
scopic appearance
of the cervix
seems to resem-
ble a retina.
(a) What is it?
(b) How is it
formed?

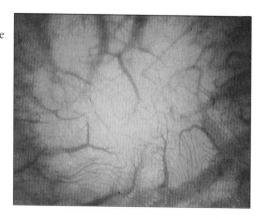

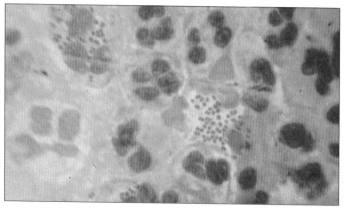

106 (a) What Gram-negative pathogens does this slide show?
(b) From what must they be differentiated?
(c) How is this achieved?

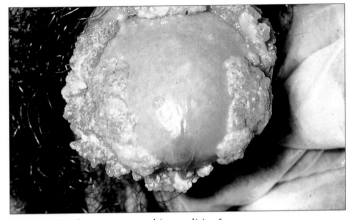

107 (a) Which virus causes this condition?
(b) In what age group do genital warts most commonly present?

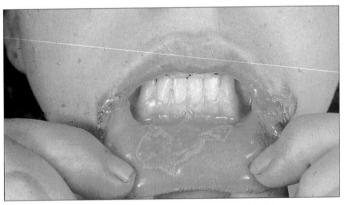

108 This lesion was found in a patient who also had hoarseness and generalised lymphadenitis.
(a) What are the lesions?
(b) When they become confluent on the fauces they are often known by what eponymous name?
(c) Why was the patient hoarse?

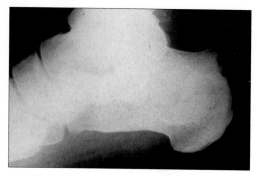

109 This radiograph of the calcaneum in a man with Reiter's disease showed this feature.
(a) What is it?
(b) What other radiological feature of the calcaneum is often seen in this condition?

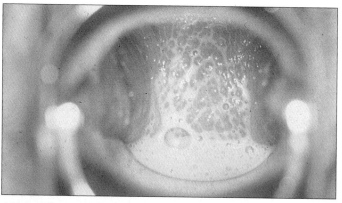

110 (a) This itchy discharge is typical of which vaginal pathogen?
(b) What symptoms would you expect in the male partner?

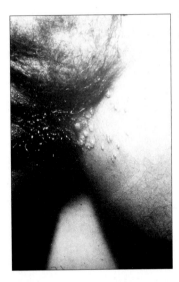

111 (a) What is the causative agent of this skin infection?
(b) How is it treated?

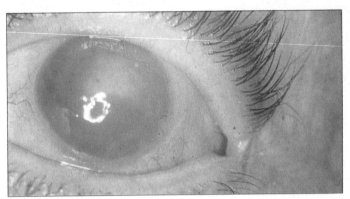

112 This 25-year-old man demonstrates the commonest late lesion of congenital syphilis.
(a) What is it?
(b) In the early stages a pink patch may be seen at the edge of the cornea. What is this due to?
(c) How is this condition thought to arise?
(d) What joint condition in congenital syphilis is also considered to arise in the same way?

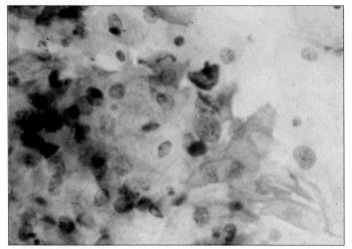

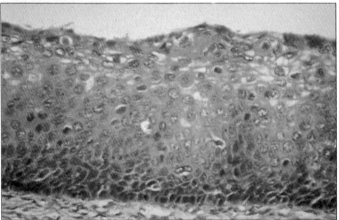

113, 114 The cytological and histological grades of CIN correspond on these two slides.
(a) What grade is shown?
(b) What is the incubation period of cervical cancer?

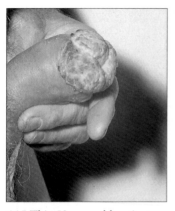

115 This 53-year-old patient did not seek medical advice for six months as he was convinced that his problem would resolve spontaneously. It was painless and there was associated bilateral lymph node enlargement.
(a) What is the condition?
(b) How is it treated?

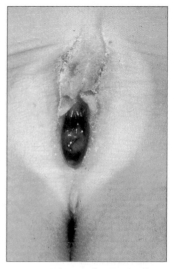

116 (a) What is this intensely pruritic pre-malignant vulval condition?
(b) Which auto-immune diseases is it occasionally linked with?

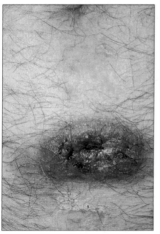

117 A 33-year-old man attended with this non-irritant lesion on his pubis. He was worried because it was discharging. He denied that it could be a sexually transmitted infection as he always used a condom. What is the lesion?

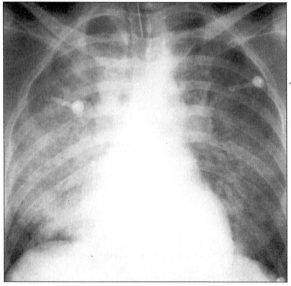

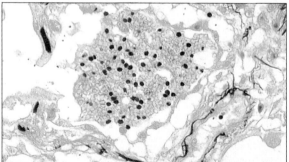

118, 119 A 22-year-old man with HIV infection presenteed with a five-week history of dry coughing, shortness of breath and, more recently, a headache. He had a mild pyrexia and was found to be hypoxic.

(a) The chest radiograph is suggestive of what condition?

(b) What is shown in his transbronchial lung biopsy that confirms the diagnosis?

(c) What other common infections may cause pulmonary disease in AIDS?

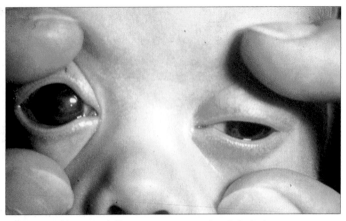

120 Complications following gonococcal ophthalmia neonatorum are severe if the infection is not promptly treated.
(a) What complication is shown?
(b) What used to be, and still is in some countries, administered to babies' eyes at birth to prevent gonorrhoea?

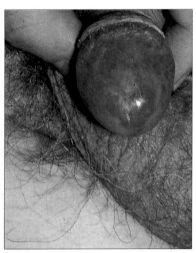

121 This chronic, slightly itchy lesion, found in a 62-year-old man, often has multiple red-pinpoint spots likened to cayenne pepper.
(a) What is it?
(b) What is found on bi-opsy?
(c) How may it be treated?

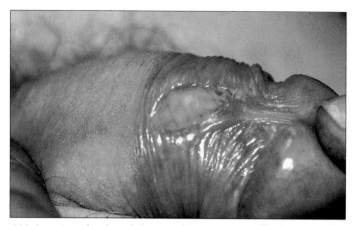

122 A patient developed this painful sore associated with slight bleeding on the second day of his honeymoon. The lesion gradually worsened.
(a) What is it?
(b) Which part of the penis is most commonly affected?

123 (a) What is this painful scrotal swelling, seen in a 22-year-old man who gave a history of a slight urethral discharge and dysuria one week earlier, which had now ceased?
(b) Which two serious conditions must be excluded from the diagnosis?
(c) List other possible causes of the condition.

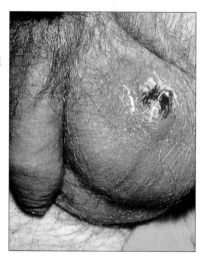

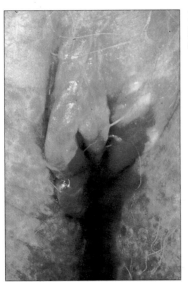

124 This woman with vulval pruritis was found to have two dermatoses. What are they?

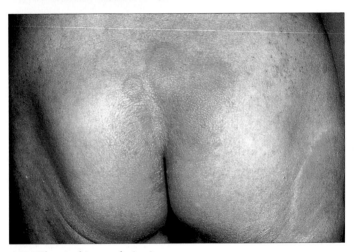

125 What is this rare lesion?

126 This patient returned to the clinic the day after commencing treatment for chlamydia. He complained of a painful, swollen prepuce and raised, erythematous lesions of the glans.
(a) What is the condition?
(b) What is the mechanism that causes it?

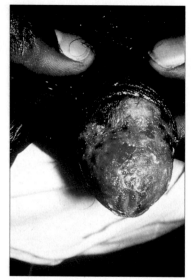

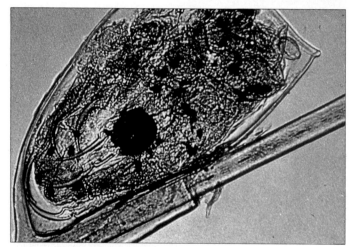

127 (a) What is the common name for this egg of a human parasite?
(b) After hatching what colour change occurs in the egg?
(c) How can the age of the egg be determined?

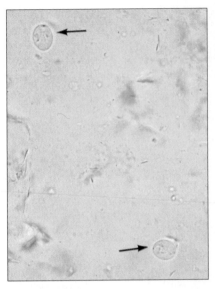

128 (a) What are these intestinal pathogens? (b) What symptoms do they usually produce? (c) How are they treated?

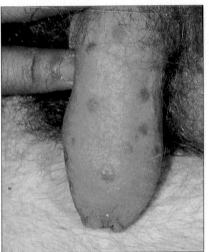

129 What is the cause of these oedematous pink papules on the penis?

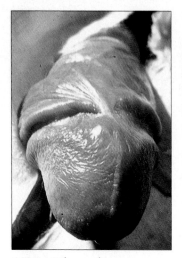

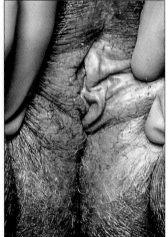

130 (a) What is this rare, insignificant complication of gonorrhoea?
(b) What predisposes to it?
(c) In parts of Africa and Asia beta-lactamase producing strains of *Neisseria gonorrhoeae* are very common. Which drugs are often used, instead of penicillin, to treat these organisms?

131 This woman had an itchy vulva and a white vaginal discharge that improved slightly with treatment. However, her symptoms rapidly recurred when therapy was discontinued.
(a) What is wrong with her?
(b) Why are the symptoms recurring?
(c) What other predisposing causes might produce a recurrence of the condition?

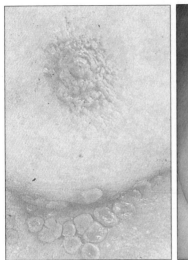
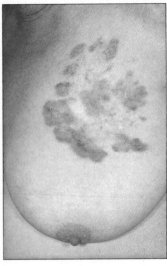

132, 133 These two women were referred to the breast clinic. Neither required surgery. Both have the same disease. What is it and which manifestations are they showing?

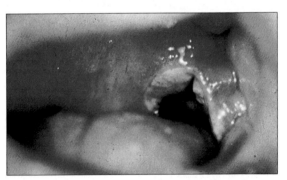

134 This patient did not return for treatment of secondary syphilis. This ulcer was found in his mouth ten years later.
(a) What is the lesion?
(b) What must be done prior to treatment?

135, 136 A 56-year-old man presented with two indurated penile ulcers of three months duration with surrounding erythema. He had right-sided, non-tender lymphadenopathy. The diagnosis of a very rare presentation of this disease was suggested by biopsy and confirmed by a positive C-ANCA test for cytoplasmic staining anti-neutrophil cytoplasmic antibodies.

(a) What did the biopsy show?
(b) What is the diagnosis?

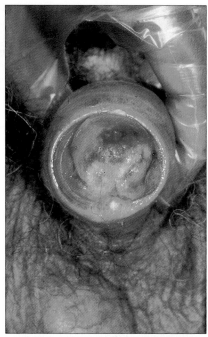

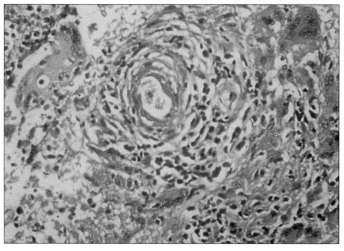

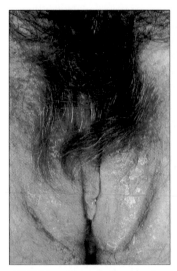 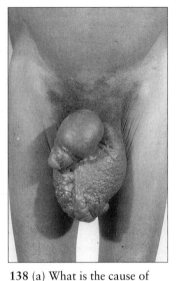

137 This patient suffers remissions and relapses of an irritant skin condition. What is it?

138 (a) What is the cause of the scrotal elephantiasis in this man with Lymphogranuloma venereum?
(b) In women, what is the condition often known as?
(c) What is the differential diagnosis of genital elephantiasis?

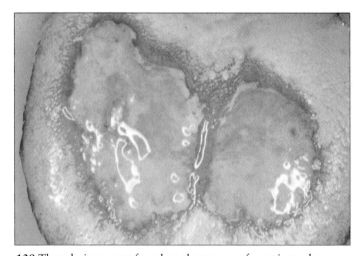

139 These lesions were found on the tongue of a patient who presented with severe fever, diarrhoea and vomiting. He also had a balanitis and a skin rash of lesions that were centrally cyanotic and erythematous at the periphery.

(a) What is the diagnosis?
(b) What agents are known to precipitate the condition?
(c) Give another name for the condition.

140 (a) What is this mouth lesion?
(b) Describe the causative agent.

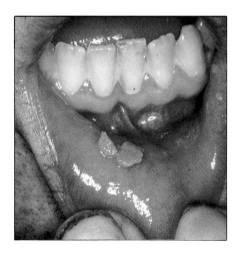

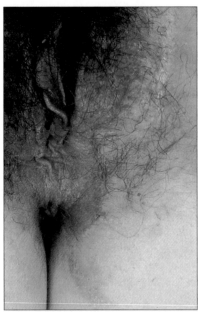

141, 142, 143 This woman suffered from small, pigmented keratotic lesions of her vulva, arm, hand and finger. She was originally thought to have an inherited autosomal dominant disease. Histology disproved this.
(a) What is this rare condition?
(b) What was the disease she was originally thought to have?

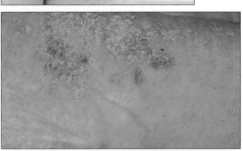

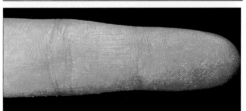

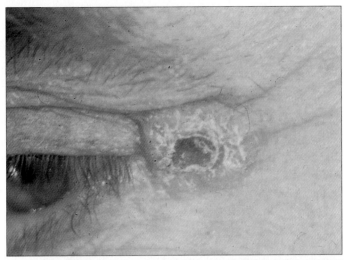

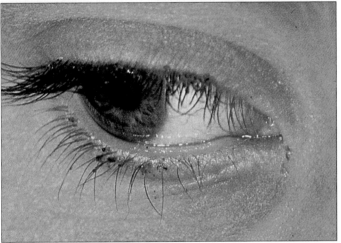

144, 145 These two patients developed different problems as a result of oral sexual practices.
(a) What is the diagnosis in each case?
(b) At what other extra-genital sites might such problems occur?

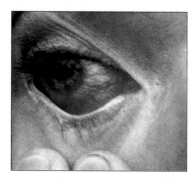

146 (a) Which condition shown is often found in recurrent seronegative reactive arthritis?
(b) Which HLA antigen is found in both spondylitis and seronegative reactive arthritis?

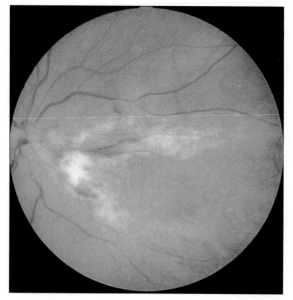

147 This patient with AIDS presented with deterioration of vision.
(a) Characteristic changes of what condition are shown?
(b) What pathological changes occur?
(c) Which are the two commonest drugs used in the treatment of this condition?
(d) What is the prognosis?

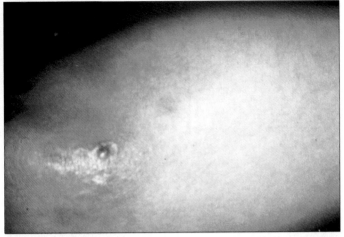

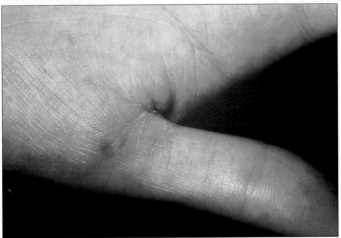

148, 149 (a) What is the cause of these lesions in a 17-year-old
girl with mild pyrexia?
(b) If severe, to where else may the condition spread?

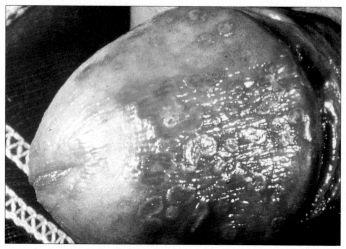

150 (a) What is this inflammatory condition?
(b) Which organisms are usually involved?

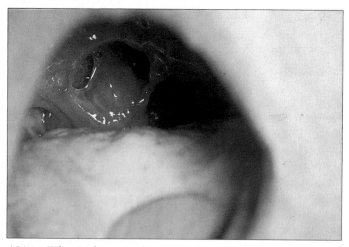

151 (a) What is shown in this picture?
(b) What is the cause?

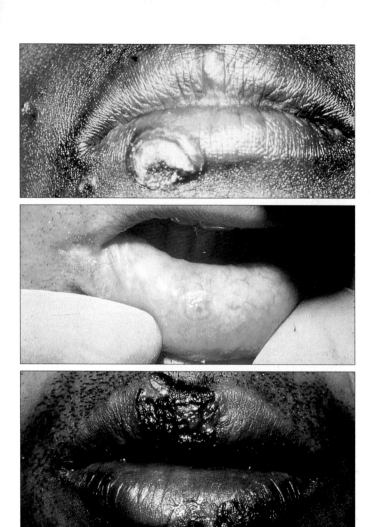

152, 153, 154 Three patients presented with similar lip lesions. The first two had painless sores and FTA-positive serology. The third patient's serology was negative but his sore was painful. The first patient was a recent immigrant from the West Indies. What is the probable diagnosis in each case?

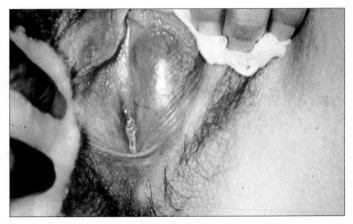

155 (a) What is this tender swelling in the lower vulval region?
(b) How is it treated?

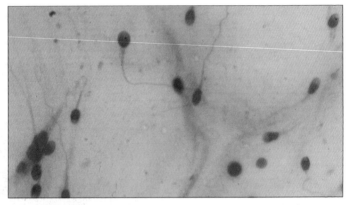

156 (a) What are shown in this picture have occasionally been attributed to be a vector for the carriage of micro-organisms from the cervix to fallopian tubes in pelvic inflammatory disease (PID).
(a) What are they?
(b) What other conditions must be eliminated in the diagnosis of PID in young women?

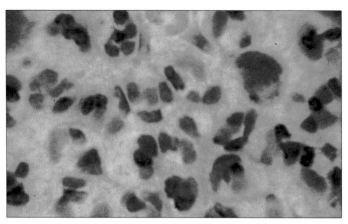

157 (a) What does this Gram-stained slide show?
(b) What are the main infective causes of this condition?

158 This 47-year-old man presented with a painless, firm-edged indurated penile ulcer and inguinal lympha-denopathy.
(a) What is the most likely diagnosis having excluded infections?
(b) What simple proce-dure would probably prevent this condition?

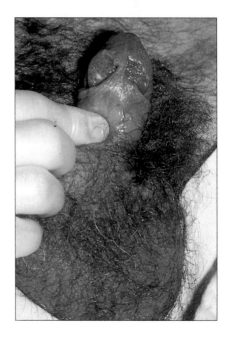

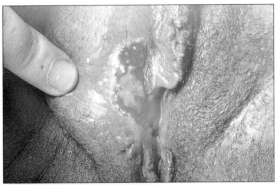

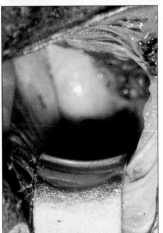

159, 160, 161
A painless vulval ulcer and granulomatous vaginal mass suggested the diagnosis in this African woman.
(a) What is the condition?
(b) How do these scrapings from the edge of the lesion confirm the diagnosis?
(c) What is the treatment of choice?

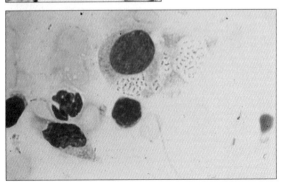

162, 163 The clinical and radiographic appearances of a neuropathic joint condition found in late syphilis are shown.
(a) What is the condition?
(b) What associated pupillary abnormality is often found that can aid the diagnosis?
(c) In what other conditions may a neuropathic joint be found?

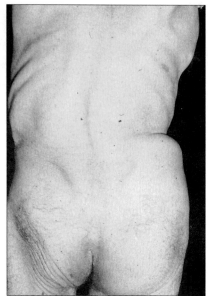

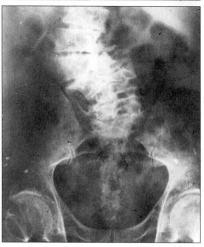

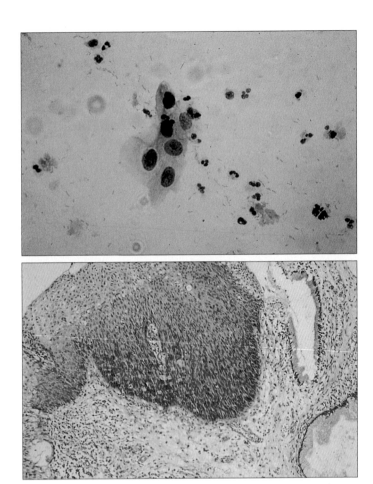

164, 165 These slides were from a patient who had a cervical biopsy following her cytology. What do they show?

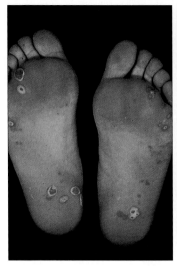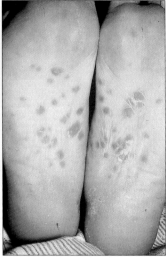

166, 167 These are rashes on the soles of two patients' feet.

(a) What is the scaly rash found in Reiter's disease called?

(b) What is the other disorder illustrated?

(c) What skin disease is associated with an arthropathy sometimes indistinguishable from Reiter's disease?

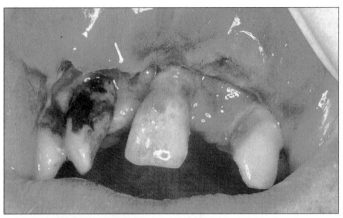

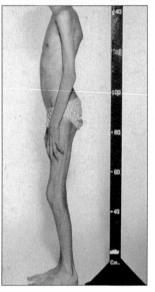

168, 169 A 29-year-old man with AIDS presented with weight loss and oral cavity disease.

(a) What are possible causes of his weight loss?

(b) What is the syndrome of wasting and severe diarrhoea, first reported in Uganda, called?

(c) What mouth lesion does he have?

(d) How is it treated?

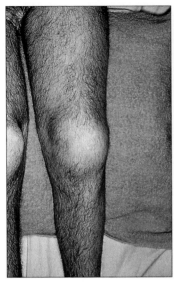

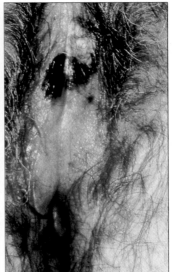

170 This patient presented with a painful, swollen knee joint that was tender and hot to the touch. His partner had gonorrhoea.

(a) What is the possible diagnosis?

(b) What would you expect to find on examination of the synovial fluid?

(c) Which drug is the treatment of choice?

171 (a) What is this pigmented lesion rarely found on the vulva?

(b) How would you differentiate it from other pigmented lesions?

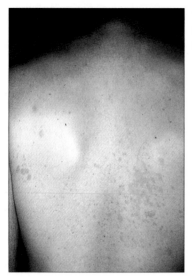

172 (a) What is this fungal skin infection?
(b) Which fungus is responsible?

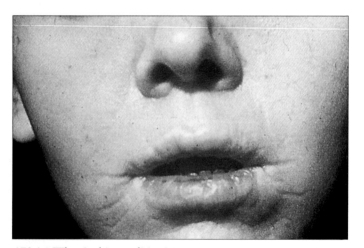

173 (a) What is this condition?
(b) What is it due to?
(c) Where else may it be found?

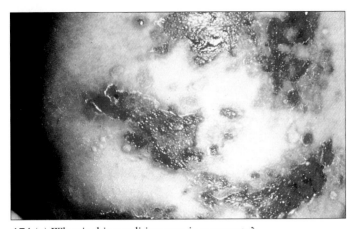

174 (a) What is this condition seen in a neonate?
(b) What main clinical manifestations are found?
(c) What sexually transmitted pathogens of viral origin may be transmitted to the neonate?

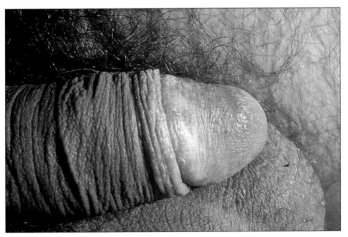

175 (a) What is the cause of the itchy rash on this man's glans?
(b) What simple test must be done to exclude systemic disease?

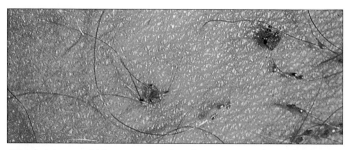

176 A 16-year-old boy presented with irritation in his pubic area together with some spots of blood on his underpants. What condition was he suffering from?

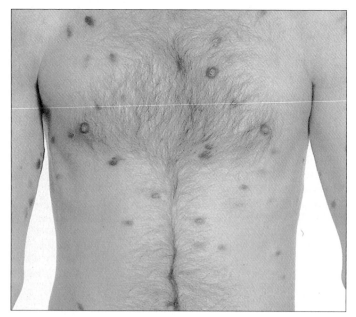

177 (a) What are these painless, purplish skin lesions in a patient with AIDS?
(b) In which risk group are they most common?
(c) What may happen if the lesions are traumatized?
(d) Prior to AIDS these lesions tended to be seen in which three patient groups?

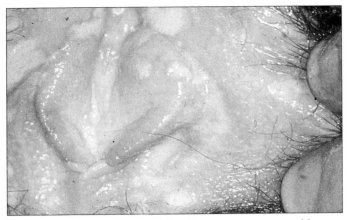

178 This girl's severe first episode of herpes was contracted by entry of the virus through lesions already present. These have a mucous appearance.

(a) What are they?

(b) List the factors that might trigger recurrent episodes of herpes.

179 This man attended with painful penile and scrotal ulcers that appeared five days after visiting a prostitute in South Africa. He subsequently developed a tender mass in the right inguinal region.

(a) What is the likely cause of these symptoms?

(b) How do the multiple ulcers on the scrotum develop?

(c) What is the common name of the inguinal mass?

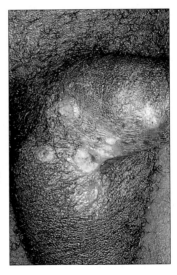

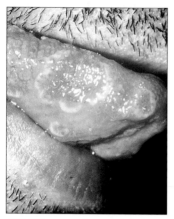

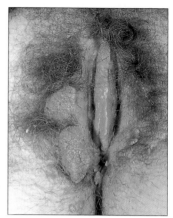

180 What are these painless erosive lesions in a patient with a painful, swollen elbow?

181 This pregnant woman attended with a rapid increase in the size and number of her genital warts.
(a) What is the mechanism thought to cause this?
(b) What is the management?

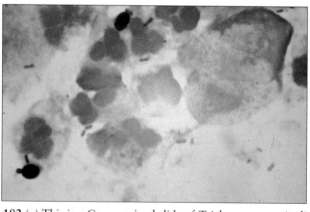

182 (a) This is a Gram-stained slide of *Trichomonas vaginalis*. How would you more easily demonstrate this organism?
(b) How many flagellae do trichomonads usually have?
(c) What are the Gram-positive organisms present?

183, 184 A 35-year-old man presented with this painless ulcer. It is biopsied by a keen young SHO and the histology is shown.
(a) What is the lesion?
(b) What does histology show?

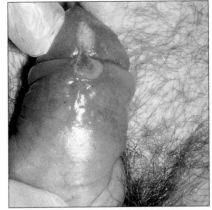

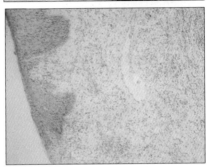

185 This patient presented with unexplained bilateral inguinal lymphadenopathy together with a slight pyrexia. He gave a history of a small red papule on his leg two weeks previously. Sexually transmitted disease was excluded.
(a) What animal was involved in his disorder?
(b) What is the causative organism?

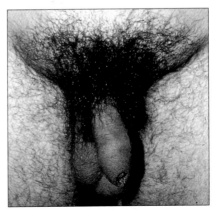

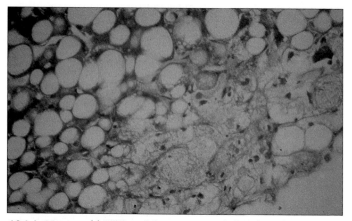

186 A 45-year-old HIV-positive man attended with malaise, weight loss and anorexia, together with discomfort in his epigastrium. Ultrasound showed diffuse liver enlargement consistent with fatty infiltration.

(a) What does histology of the liver biopsy show?
(b) What is the causative organism?
(c) How is it treated?
(d) What can happen if untreated?

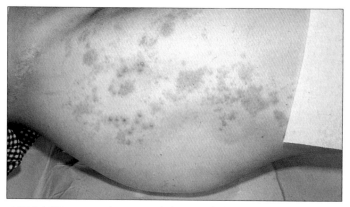

187 (a) What organism caused this painful, unilateral skin rash?
(b) What drug is the treatment of choice?

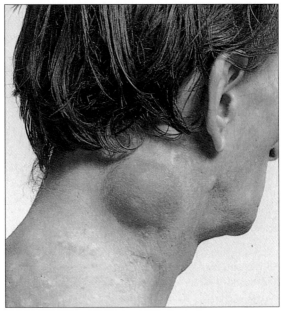

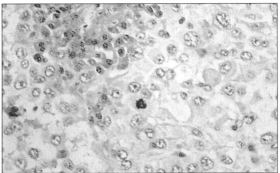

188, 189 A 34-year-old AIDS patient presented with this cervical swelling.

(a) What is the likely cause?

(b) What does histology of the lesion show?

(c) Where in the body do these lesions more commonly occur?

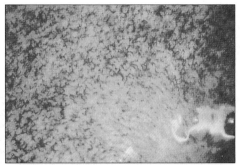

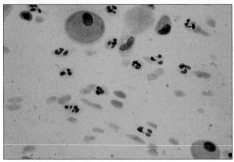

190, 191 These pictures illustrate the colposcopic appearance and cytology of a woman presenting with dyspareunia and bloodstained vaginal discharge.
(a) What is the diagnosis?
(b) How is the condition treated?

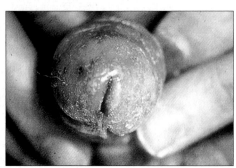

192 This teenager complained of pain under his foreskin.
(a) What is the cause of this?
(b) What advice would you give him?

193 This is a colposcopic appearance of vulval intra-epithelial-neoplasia grade 3. What HPV type is commonly found in these lesions?

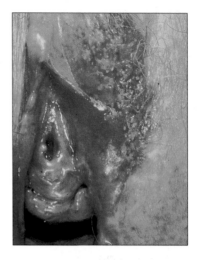

194 (a) What is the cause of this non-irritating rash?
(b) What is the differential diagnosis?
(c) What blood test will quickly confirm the diagnosis?
(d) Is the blood test always positive in this condition?

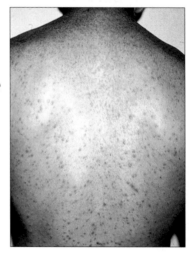

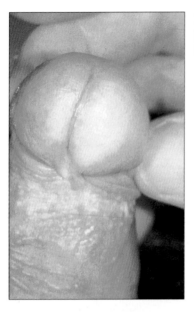

195 What are the slightly pruritic areas on this man's penis?

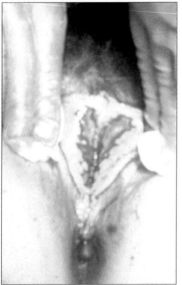

196 This patient was using a well-known proprietary antiseptic undiluted, subsequently developing this vulval lesion. What is it?

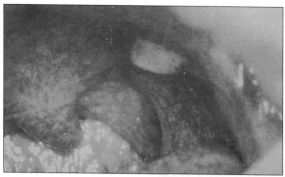

197, 198, 199 Six weeks after having sexual intercourse with a prostitute in Nairobi, this patient presented with tiredness, fever, maculopapular rash, retro-orbital pain, lymphadenopathy and a sore, ulcerated throat. He did not have syphilis.
(a) What is the probable cause of his symptoms?
(b) What other symptoms sometimes occur?
(c) What is the usual differential diagnosis?

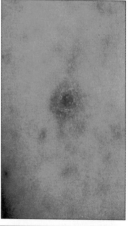

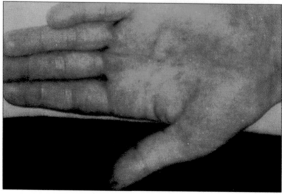

200 (a) What percentage of men with perianal condyloma acuminata have associated warts in the anal canal?
(b) What is the incubation period of genital warts?

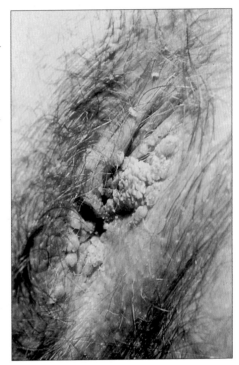

ANSWERS

1 Multiple sebaceous cysts.

2 (a) Primary syphilis.
(b) Chancre.
(c) Firmly enlarged, mobile, discrete, painless inguinal lymph nodes.

3 (a) Gonococcal urethritis.
(b) Chlamydial and non-gonococcal urethritis, trichomoniasis, herpes and discharge secondary to lesions in the urethra (e.g. warts). Occasionally, discharge secondary to prostatitis or upper urinary tract lesions may be seen.

4 (a) Non-sclerosing lymphangitis due to oedema.
(b) Non-specific trauma.
(c) None. It usually resolves spontaneously.

5 (a) Molluscum contagiosum.
(b) AIDS.

6 (a) Osteoperiostitis of the tibia.
(b) Sabre tibia.
(c) Congenital syphilis and yaws.

7 Normal coronal papillae (hirsutes papillaris penis). They are more prominent in some individuals.

8 (a) Behçets disease.
(b) The Mediterranean, the Middle East and Japan.
(c) Syphilis, herpes and malignancy.

9 (a) *Sarcoptes scabiei,* which causes scabies.
(b) Stratum corneum.

10 (a) Hairy leukoplakia, which is thought to be unique to HIV-infected patients.
(b) Epstein–Barr virus.

11 (a) Herpes zoster.
(b) Usually unilateral in herpes zoster as opposed to bilateral in herpes simplex infection.

12 (a) Pseudomycelia and spores of *Candida albicans.*
(b) At pH 5.4 on Sabouraud's medium.

13 (a) Secondary syphilis.
(b) Soles of the feet and the face.

14, 15 (a) Reactive arthritis of Reiter's disease.
(b) Circinate balanitis.

16 (a) Chlamydia inclusion in tissue-culture cell.
(b) Ophthalmia neonatorum and pneumonia. It also predisposes to pre-term delivery.

17, 18 (a) A CIN grade 3 smear with greatly enlarged, monomorphic dyskaryotic nuclei and very little cytoplasm.
(b) Carcinoma of the cervix.

19 The 'school of fish' appearance of *Haemophilus ducreyi.*

20 (a) Hutchinson's Teeth. The permanent incisors, most commonly the upper central, are affected. Due to defective development of the medial tooth buds, the teeth converge to the cutting edge like the sides of a peg. They are occasionally notched.
(b) Congenital syphilis.
(c) Moon's (Mulberry) molars. The first lower molars are underdeveloped with poorly enameled cusps and a dome-shaped biting surface. They are very prone to caries.

21 (a) 'Saxaphone' penis.
(b) Minor pyogenic infection.

22 (a) Ophthalmia neonatorum.
(b) *Neisseria gonorrhoeae*, *Chlamydia trachomatis*, *Haemophilus influenzae*, staphylococci and streptococci.
(c) Isolate the baby. Administer intramuscular penicillin if the causative agent is gonococcal, erythromycin syrup if chlamydial. Undertake local saline bathing, and examine and treat the infant's parents if necessary.

23 (a) Koilocytes (cells with large, clear cytoplasmic vacuoles). The periphery of the cytoplasm is dense and the nuclei are irregular and hyperchromatic.
(b) They are regarded as pathognomonic of warts virus infection.

24 (a) *Treponema pallidum*.
(b) Dark-field microscopy.

25 (a) Bilateral fallopian tubal blockage.
(b) Pelvic inflammatory disease, usually caused by gonorrhoea or chlamydia.
(c) Laparoscopy.

26 Paget's disease, an intra-epidermal carcinoma.

27 Lymphoid interstitial pneumonia.

28 Restoration of immune defence mechanisms and full maturation of the vaginal epithelium following the removal of the mainly progestogenic effect of the pill.

29 (a) *Trichomonas vaginalis.*
(b) Metronidazole.

30 (a) Herpes genitalis.
(b) Culture of serum from the lesions. Exclude syphilis by dark-field examination.

31 (a) Condylomata lata.
(b) The secondary stage of syphilis.
(c) In moist areas such as the groin, perineum and the perianal area, the axillae and under the breasts.
(d) Penicillin.

32 (a) Cervicitis.
(b) Gonorrhoea, chlamydia and non-specific infection, herpes and trichomoniasis.

33 (a) A gumma of tertiary syphilis.
(b) A wash-leather.

(c) Gummas tend to involve mainly the proximal, lateral lower leg as opposed to varicose ulcers, which involve the distal, medial lower leg.

34 (a) Herpes simplex virus.
(b) The trigeminal ganglion in oral infections. The sacral dorsal root ganglia (S2-S4) in genital infections.

35 (a) Conjunctivitis with urethritis and arthritis.
(b) One per cent.
(c) Dysentery.

36 (a) Podophyllin resin.
(b) Podophyllotoxin (the active ingredient of podophyllin), trichloracetic acid, cryotherapy (nitrous oxide cryoprobe, liquid nitrogen), electrocautery and surgical excision in some cases.

37, 38 Burrows of scabies.

39 (a) 'Violin string' adhesions between the anterior surface of the liver and the adjacent abdominal wall.
(b) Fitz-Hugh-Curtis syndrome. This is an acute perihepatitis that often follows pelvic inflammatory disease.
(c) *Chlamydia trachomatis* or *Neisseria gonorrhoeae*.
(d) Liver and gall bladder disease, pleurisy, pneumonia ands perforated peptic ulcer.

40 (a) Oesophageal candidiasis, probably extending from the buccal cavity.
(b) Ketoconazole or fluconazole.

(c) There is a slight risk of liver damage with keto-conazole but this risk is acceptable in AIDS patients.

(d) *Herpes simplex*, cytomegalovirus and aphthous ulceration.

41 Endometriosis of the cervix.

42 (a) Chancroid.
(b) *Haemophilus ducreyi*.
(c) Culture.

43 (a) Tinea cruris.
(b) *Trichophyton rubrum* and *Epidermophyton floccosum*. Often also found on the feet.
(c) Erythrasma, candidiasis, psoriasis and intertrigo.

44 (a) Vaginitis due to *Candida albicans*, commonly known as thrush.
(b) A thick, white discharge, dysuria and vulval or perianal pruritis.

45 (a) Auto-inoculation.
(b) The buttocks, limbs, eyes and lips.

46 Multinucleate giant cells suggestive of herpes virus infection.

47 HPV 6, 11, 16, 18 and occasionally HPV 33.

48 (a) 'Clue cells' (epithelial cells covered with the Gram-variable cocci of *Gardnerella vaginalis*).
(b) Bacterial vaginosis.

(c) If symptomatic, with metronidazole. Clindamycin cream is useful if systemic therapy is not indicated. There is no evidence to suggest that treatment of the male partner diminishes the recurrence rate.

49 (a) She has the vulval lesions of secondary syphilis. The patchy, 'moth-eaten' alopecia is an occasional manifestation of this stage of the disease.
(b) Her hair will grow normally again after resolution or treatment of syphilis.

50 (a) Balanitis xerotica obliterans.
(b) Phimosis.
(c) Steroid creams may help in the early stages, but circumcision is usually required eventually.
(d) Lichen sclerosus et atrophicus.

51 (a) Chronic superficial glossitis.
(b) It is premalignant and biopsy should be performed if ulceration occurs.

52 Recurrent *Herpes simplex* infection of the urethral meatus.

53, 54, 55 (a) Behçets disease.
(b) Erythema nodosum skin lesions, erythema multiforme, arthritis, GI-tract symptoms, CNS involvement and recurrent oral ulcers.

56 (a) Primary syphilis.
(b) Protoscopy should be carried out as there is often a lesion in the anal canal.
(c) Anal fissure.

57 (a) The protozoan *Cryptosporidium*.
(b) Cytomegalovirus, *Mycobacterium avium-intracellulare* and *Isospora belli*.

58 (a) Basal cell carcinoma (epithelioma).
(b) Chimney sweeps, coal-gas workers and mule spinners.

59 (a) Pityriasis rosea.
(b) The herald patch, which typically precedes the main rash.
(c) None is required as it usually clears spontaneously in about six weeks.

60 He has a contact dermatitis.

61 (a) Secondary infection.
(b) A cell-mediated reaction caused by sensitization to the mite.

62 (a) Yaws.
(b) Endemic syphilis (Africa, the Middle East, Australia), known as bejel in Iraq and njovera in Zimbabwe. Pinta (Central and South America).

63 Eczema of the penis.

64, 65, 66 (a) Invasive squamous carcinoma of the cervix.
(b) Malignant cells showing pleomorphism and lack of organized relationship or structure.
(c) Papanicolaou.

67 Cutaneous gumma of tertiary syphilis causing 'tissue-paper scarring'.

68 Ulcer of Behçet's disease causing the star-shaped 'splash' fibrosis.

69 (a) Urethral stricture.
(b) Gonorrhoea.

70 (a) Lymphogranuloma venereum.
(b) Syphilis, herpes, Donovanosis, chancroid, filariasis and cat-scratch disease.

71 A cervical polyp.

72 Tinea infection.

73 (a) *Chlamydia trachomatis* conjunctivitis showing typical follicular lesions.
(b) Trachoma.

74 (a) Primary syphilis.
(b) Between nine and 90 days. On average, 21 days.
(c) An acute febrile reaction within hours of starting treatment, sometimes with exacerbation of skin and mucosal lesions. There should be no recurrence with subsequent treatment.
(d) Jarisch-Herxheimer reaction.

75 Haemangioma.

76 Adenocarcinoma in-situ.

77 (a) Proctitis.

(b) Gonorrhoea, chlamydia, herpes, syphilis, warts, helminthic infections, e.g. threadworms (*Enterobius vermicularis*), lymphogranuloma venereum, trauma, e.g. caused by foreign bodies, 'fisting', medications, e.g. podophyllin and for inflammatory bowel diseases like Crohn's disease.

78 (a) Lactobacilli.
(b) To maintain vaginal acidity, thus inhibiting the growth of most other pathogens.
(c) They produce lactic acid from mucosal glycogen.

79 (a) *Toxoplasma gondii.*
(b) Brain abscess.

80 (a) A nodulo-cutaneous gumma of tertiary syphilis.
(b) Penicillin.

81, 82 (a) Lichen planus.
(b) Wickham's striae.

83 (a) Erythroplasia of Queyrat.
(b) It is premalignant; biopsy shows the changes of an intra-epidermal carcinoma.

84 (a) Oedema of the prepuce.
(b) Retention of urine, secondary infection, encephalitis and aseptic meningitis.

85 (a) *Pthirus pubis* (crab louse), which causes pediculosis pubis.
(b) Two forms of *Pediculus humanus*, one causing pediculosis capitis and the other causing pediculosis corporis.

(c) The body louse may transmit typhus or relapsing fever.

86 (a) Framboesioma of secondary yaws.
(b) *Treponema pertenue*.
(c) By close childhood contact in poor hygienic and social conditions. Occasionally to previously uninfected adults from an infected child.

87 (a) Peyronie's disease.
(b) Plaques in penis.
(c) Dupuytren's contracture.

88 Lichen sclerosus et atrophicus.

89, 90 (a) Aortic aneurysm. The mass has eroded the sternum and extended onto the chest wall. The radiograph shows an aneurysm of the ascending aorta.
(b) A pulsatile mass.
(c) Aortitis, aortic incompetence, coronary ostial stenosis.

91, 92 Cervical-wart virus infection.

93 Microscopic examination of skin scrapings immersed in a drop of twenty-per-cent potassium hydroxide. This destroys other tissue, enabling fungal elements to be seen.

94 (a) Prepubertal vulvovaginitis may be due to infection with gonorrhoea, chlamydia, candida or skin conditions.

(b) Sexual contact (not always admitted), non-sexual contact with infected adults, accidental transmission from towels or rectal thermometers. The possibility of sexual abuse should never be forgotten.

95 (a) Hypospadias.
(b) Para-urethral pigmented naevus.

96 (a) Dark-field microscopy of serum from the lesion. The IgM fraction of the FTA (fluorescent treponemal antibody) blood test is useful, as this large molecule cannot be transferred across the placenta. Thus, if present, infection is indicated. It is not completely reliable however, and serology at six months will rule out passive transfer of maternal antibodies.
(b) Yes, in early congenital syphilis only, usually at birth.
(c) There is no primary chancre in congenital syphilis. The transplacental infection corresponds to the secondary stage of acquired syphilis.

97 Periurethral abscess.

98 (a) Urethral meatal warts.
(b) Urethritis, trauma, carcinoma and haematuria.

99 (a) Median-raphe sinus.
(b) Yes. Often infections such as gonorrhoea, as in this case, enter the blind sinus causing it to discharge.

100 (a) AIDS.
(b) *Herpes simplex*.

101, 102 (a) Lymphogranuloma vereneum.

(b) *Chlamydia trachomatis* serovars L1, L2 and L3.

(c) Groove sign. Indentation of bubo by the inguinal ligament.

103 (a) Paraphimosis.

(b) When the constricting ring of the prepuce prevents replacement following retraction.

(c) Early: manual reduction. Late: surgical division of band and circumcision.

104 (a) Choroido-retinitis.

(b) 'Pepper and salt' fundus.

105 (a) A Nabothian follicle.

(b) By mucous secreted by columnar cells in the transformation zone forming a retention cyst.

106 (a) *Neisseria gonorrhoeae.*

(b) Other *Neisseria* species both pathogenic, e.g. *Neisseria meningitidis* and non-pathogenic, e.g. *Neisseria pharyngis.*

(c) By different carbohydrate utilization tests on culture, and monoclonal antibody tests.

107 (a) Human papillomavirus (HPV).

(b) Twenty to 24 years of age.

108 (a) Mucous patches of secondary syphilis.

(b) 'Snail-track' ulcers.

(c) Due to lesions involving the vocal cords.

109 (a) Erosion of the Achilles tendon insertion.

(b) A periosteal calcaneal spur at the plantar fascia attachment.

110 (a) *Trichomonas vaginalis.*
(b) Usually none but occasionally there is a slight urethral discharge.

111 (a) A pox virus (molluscum contagiosum).
(b) Pricking the lesion with phenol or trichloracetic acid, or by electro-cautery.

112 (a) Interstitial keratitis.
(b) The 'salmon patch' is due to corneal vascularisation.
(c) An immunological reaction as opposed to direct effect of the infection.
(d) Clutton's joints. A chronic painless synovitis.

113, 114 (a) Grade CIN 2.
(b) For squamous cell tumours usually 10 to 15 years. A faster-growing, small-cell type of glandular origin, with very little pre-invasive stage, arising from the endocervical canal, is becoming commoner in younger women.

115 (a) Squamous-cell carcinoma.
(b) Radiotherapy, preceded by partial excision of the tumour if it does not involve the shaft.

116 (a) Lichen sclerosus et atrophicus.
(b) Thyroid disease and pernicious anaemia.

117 A 'condom' chancre of primary syphilis. The lesion is at the base of the penis or pubic area as the rest of the penis is protected.

118, 119 (a) *Pneumocystis carinii* pneumonia with fluffy interstitial shadowing spreading from the hilum.

(b) *Pneumocystis carinii* in the intra-alveolar exudate.

(c) Cytomegalovirus, *Legionella*, *Mycobacterium tuberculosis*, *Mycobacterium avium-intracellulare*, pyogenic bacteria (e.g. *Haemophilus influenzae*, *Streptococcus pneumoniae*).

120 (a) Corneal opacity, following keratitis, causing blindness.

(b) One-per-cent silver nitrate solution.

121 (a) Plasma-cell balanitis of Zoon.

(b) On biopsy, dense infiltration with plasma cells, probably non-specific, together with epidermal atrophy and wide separation of typical lozenge-shaped keratinocytes, is revealed.

(c) Symptoms may be controlled by steroids but complete cure is obtained by circumcision.

122 (a) Traumatic ulcer, due to over-vigorous sexual intercourse.

(b) The frenum.

123 (a) Epididymitis secondary to gonorrhoea or non-gonococcal urethritis. In this patient the infection has spread to the testes and rupture through the scrotal wall is threatened.

(b) Torsion of the testis and testicular tumour.

(c) Secondary to urinary tract infection. Other infections, i.e. mumps, tuberculosis, brucellosis, meningitis, filariasis and mycoses. Occasionally presents in Behçet's disease.

124 Lichen planus and lichen sclerosus.

125 An annular gumma of tertiary syphilis.

126 (a) Fixed-drug eruption due to tetracycline.
(b) Probably an immunologically mediated process.

127 (a) Nit (of crab louse).
(b) It turns white.
(c) The egg, being attached to the hair, moves distally as the hair grows.

128 (a) The protozoan *Giardia lamblia*.
(b) Flatulence, nausea, abdominal pain and diarrhoea. Occasionally asymptomatic.
(c) Metronidazole.

129 Scabies.

130 (a) Tysonitis. Infection of the parafrenal glands of Tyson.
(b) Poor hygiene. A long prepuce.
(c) Ciprofloxacin, spectinomycin and cefuroxime.

131 (a) Vulvitis due to *Candida albicans*.
(b) Uncontrolled diabetes mellitus.
(c) Recurrence could be due to pregnancy, antibiotic therapy, immunosuppression or reinfection from an untreated partner.

132 Condylomata lata of secondary syphilis.

133 Gumma of tertiary syphilis.

134 (a) Tonsillar gumma of tertiary syphilis.
(b) Biopsy. Gummata of this area are prone to malignant change.

135, 136 (a) Extensive necrosis with vasculitis and multinucleate giant cells within venous walls.
(b) Wegener's granulomatosis, a syndrome characterized by granulomatous vasculitis of the respiratory tract and glomerulonephritis.

137 Psoriasis.

138 (a) Chronic lymphatic oedema.
(b) Esthiomene.
(c) Filariasis, Donovanosis, tuberculosis, parasites or fungi.

139 (a) Erythema multiforme.
(b) Drug sensitivity, *Herpes simplex*, lymphogranuloma venereum and *Treponema pallidum*.
(c) Stevens–Johnson syndrome.

140 (a) Condylomata acuminata (warts) transmitted by oral sex.
(b) The human papilloma virus, an icosahedral, DNA virus.

141, 142, 143 (a) Inflammatory linear naevus.
(b) Darier's disease.

144 , 145 The first patient is suffering from a primary chancre on the outer canthus of the eye. Extragenital chancres can be found on the lips, tonsils, nipples and fingers. In the second patient, there is pediculosis pubis infection of the eyelashes. Extra-genital P. pubis can also occur on the thighs, trunk and axillae.

146 (a) Uveitis.
(b) HLA-B27.

147 (a) Cytomegalovirus retinitis.
(b) Retinal vasculitis leading to areas of infarction.
(c) Ganciclovir, phosphonoformate.
(d) Unless treated, progressive impairment of visual acuity spreading to both eyes will occur, which may result in blindness.

148, 149 (a) Typical skin lesions and arthralgia of disseminated gonococcal infection.
(b) To the heart (endocarditis) and meninges.

150 (a) Erosive balanitis.
(b) Fusiforms and non-specific spirochaetes.

151 (a) Perforation of the palate.
(b) Gummatous destruction in congenital syphilis.

152 Primary yaws.

153 Primary syphilis.

154 Recurrent herpes simplex.

155 (a) Abscess of Bartholin's gland.
(b) Antibiotics if early, but in late cases and to prevent

recurrence, surgical treatment by marsupialization is necessary.

156 (a) Spermatozoa.
(b) Ectopic pregnancy, ovarian cyst, endometriosis, appendicitis or abortion of pregnancy.

157 (a) Polymorphs, which in the absence of specific infection signify non-gonococcal urethritis.
(b) *Chlamydia trachomatis*, *Ureaplasma urealyticum*. *Mycoplasma genitalium*. One third of cases have no known cause.

158 (a) Ulcerative squamous-cell carcinoma.
(b) Circumcision in first few days after birth.

159, 160, 161 (a) Donovanosis.
(b) They show the 'safety pin' appearance, which is due to bipolar staining of Donovan bodies (*Calymnatobacterium granulomatis*) in mononuclear cells.
(c) Cotrimoxazole or tetracycline.

162, 163 (a) Charcot's arthropathy.
(b) Argyll–Robertson pupils. Small, non-reactive to light but reactive to accommodation.
(c) Syringomyelia, diabetes mellitus and spinal cord injury.

164 This shows a CIN grade **1** smear with mild dyskaryosis.

165 The patient's biopsy shows that the lesion is in fact worse (CIN grade 3). There is a loss of stratification, pleomorphism, hyperchromatic nuclei and mitotic figures.

166, 167 (a) Keratoderma blenorrhagica.
(b) Secondary syphilis.
(c) Psoriasis.

168, 169 (a) Anorexia due to gastrointestinal tract disease and diarrhoea, possible malabsorption and psychological problems.
(b) 'Slim' disease.
(c) Severe gingivitis with gum recession.
(d) Penicillin or metronidazole and good oral hygiene.

170 (a) An acute gonococcal septic arthritis.
(b) A purulent fluid with the presence of *Neisseria gonorrhoeae*.
(c) Penicillin. Most cases are highly sensitive to this.

171 (a) Malignant melanoma.
(b) Excision biopsy is the safest method.

172 (a) Tinea versicolor.
(b) *Malassezia furfur*.

173 (a) Rhagades of congenital syphilis.
(b) Scars from fissuring during the papular eruption in early syphilis.
(c) Around the nares and anus.

174 (a) Neonatal herpes.
(b) Skin lesions, encephalitis and meningitis.

(c) Herpes simplex, cytomegalovirus, hepatitis B virus, human papilloma virus and HIV.

175 (a) Balanitis due to *Candida albicans*.
(b) Test for glycosuria to exclude diabetes mellitus.

176 Pediculosis pubis.

177 (a) Kaposi's sarcoma.
(b) Homosexual men.
(c) Being a vascular tumour profuse bleeding can occur.
(d) (i) Elderly, predominantly male Jews or East Europeans.
(ii) Africans (endemic).
(iii) Patients on immunosuppressive therapy.

178 (a) Mucous patches of secondary syphilis.
(b) Stress, illness, menstruation, trauma and ultra-violet light.

179 (a) Chancroid.
(b) Auto-inoculation.
(c) Bubo.

180 Tongue lesions of Reiter's disease.

181 (a) Alterations in cell-mediated immune responses occurring in pregnancy.
(b) Wait until the puerperium, when the warts reduce in size and become more amenable to treatment by the usual methods.

182 (a) By phase-contrast or dark-field microscopy together with culture.
(b) Four.
(c) Budding yeast spores, probably *Candida albicans*.

183, 184 (a) Chancre of primary syphilis.
(b) Endarteritis obliterans, capillary proliferation and perivascular infiltration with plasma cells and histiocytes.

185 (a) A cat. He has cat-scratch disease.
(b) It has been previously linked with *Afipia felis* but recent work suggests that it may possibly be caused by *Rochalimaea henselae*.

186 (a) Bacillary peliosis hepatis.
(b) *Rochalimaea henselae*.
(c) Erythromycin.
(d) Pancytopenia, hyperkinesis or rupture of the liver.

187 (a) *Varicella zoster* virus.
(b) Acyclovir.

188, 189 (a) Enlarged posterior cervical lymph node.
(b) Non-Hodgkins high-grade histiocyte lymphoma.
(c) Gastrointestinal tract, central nervous system, bone marrow and muco-cutaneous tissues.

190, 191 (a) Atrophic vaginitis in a post-menopausal woman.
(b) Hormone replacement therapy with oestrogens.

192 (a) Poor genital hygiene causing sub-preputial adhesions.

(b) Retraction of prepuce and saline bathing once to twice daily.

193 HPV 16.

194 (a) Secondary syphilis. Maculo-papular rash.

(b) Pityriasis rosea, lichen planus, chickenpox, scabies, psoriasis, tinea, measles, drug rashes, infectious mononucleosis, HIV seroconversion rash or erythema multiforme,

(c) VDRL, TPHA, FTA. serological tests.

(d) Generally yes but in some HIV-positive patients with symptoms, the blood tests for syphilis may remain negative for up to three weeks after the rash appears.

195 Lichen sclerosus et atrophicus.

196 A chemical burn due to the use of undiluted antiseptic.

197, 198, 199 (a) Seroconversion illness of HIV infection.

(b) Encephalitis, transient myelopathy.

(c) Secondary syphilis, pityriasis rosea, rubella or infectious mononucleosis.

200 (a) Over fifty per cent.

(b) Three weeks to eight months. On average, three months.

INDEX

Numbers refer to the number shared
by the illustration, question and
answer